THE JOURNEY TO LIFELONG DENTAL WELLNESS

APOLONIA SMILES

THE JOURNEY TO LIFELONG DENTAL WELLNESS

CONTENT

INTRODUCTION

Greetings from Dr. Asker

Dentistry is more than just a profession to me—it's a family legacy and a lifelong mission. As a proud second-generation dentist, this guide reflects both my personal passion and professional commitment. Growing up in a family deeply rooted in dentistry, I witnessed firsthand the powerful impact that compassionate, skilled care can have on patients' lives. My journey in dentistry has been shaped by a commitment to excellence and a desire to continually improve. I am driven to stay at the forefront of advancements in the field and always seek new ways to enhance patient care, ensuring that each person receives the best treatment possible.

The Evolution of Dental Care

To appreciate where we are today, it's essential to understand how far we have come. The evolution of dental care is a remarkable journey from rudimentary practices to the sophisticated, evidence-based approaches we employ now.

In ancient times, dental care was rudimentary at best. Early civilizations used rudimentary tools and techniques. The Egyptians, for instance, employed a mixture of herbs and minerals for treating dental issues, and the Greeks began to formalize some dental practices around 500 BCE. Fast forward to the 19th century, when dentistry began to emerge as a recognized profession. The invention of the dental drill, the development of anesthesia, and the advent of X-rays marked significant milestones. These innovations laid the groundwork for modern dentistry, transforming it from a craft into a science.

In recent decades, we've witnessed tremendous advancements in dental technology and practices. From digital imaging and laser treatments to advanced materials and techniques in preventive care, the field has evolved to offer more effective and comfortable treatments than ever before. The integration of evidence-based practices and patient-centered care has become the gold standard, ensuring that treatments are not only effective but also tailored to the individual needs of each patient.

The Philosophy Behind Lifelong Dental Wellness

Dental care is not just about fixing problems when they arise—it's about preventing them in the first place. True dental wellness is a lifelong journey, one that involves daily habits, smart choices, and a partnership with a dental care provider you trust. It extends beyond brushing and flossing; it encompasses nutrition, lifestyle, and even the way we manage stress. This book is designed to guide you through that journey, helping you understand the deeper connections between oral health and overall health while providing actionable steps to keep your smile strong for life.

What Sets Apolonia Smiles Apart

At Apolonia Smiles, we believe that dentistry should be proactive, patient-centered, and deeply rooted in education. Our approach is built on personalized care, cutting-edge technology, and a commitment to making every visit as comfortable and stress-free as possible. Whether it's through advanced preventive care, state-of-the-art restorative treatments, or patient education, we strive to equip our patients with everything they need to maintain optimal oral health. While this book serves as a comprehensive guide to dental wellness, it also reflects the philosophy we bring to our practice every day.

The Goal of This Book

My goal in writing this guide is to empower you with the knowledge and tools needed to take charge of your lifelong dental health. I believe that understanding the principles of good oral care and incorporating them into your daily life can have a profound impact on your overall well-being. This book is designed to be more than just a guide; it is a comprehensive resource aimed at helping you navigate your dental health journey with confidence.

Throughout these pages, you will find practical advice, scientifically backed information, and actionable steps to achieve and maintain optimal dental wellness. Whether you are seeking to prevent dental issues, manage existing conditions, or simply enhance your oral hygiene routine, this book offers strategies and insights to support you at every stage.

As you turn the pages ahead, I invite you to view your oral health through a new lens—not just as a necessity, but as an essential part of your overall well-being. Let this book be your companion in making informed decisions about your oral health and in cultivating habits that will serve you well for years to come. Together, we can make a significant difference in not only achieving but also maintaining a healthier, more vibrant smile.

With warm regards and unwavering commitment,

Hussam Asker, DDS

CHAPTER

1

THE FOUNDATION OF A HEALTHY SMILE

Your Mouth: A Gateway to Better Health

When most people think about oral health, they focus on keeping their teeth white, straight, and free from cavities. However, the health of your mouth impacts much more than just your smile. Your mouth is a vital gateway to your overall health, playing a significant role in how your body functions, ages, and fights disease.

While it's essential to brush and floss regularly to prevent cavities and gum disease, it's equally important to understand how maintaining a healthy mouth can influence the rest of your body. Oral health isn't just about your teeth—it reflects your body's well-being as a whole. Taking care of your mouth can improve not only your smile but also your long-term health, helping you live a healthier, more vibrant life.

What happens in your mouth affects how you feel, how your body fights disease, and even how you age. By prioritizing your oral health now, you can avoid problems later and improve your overall wellness for years to come.

The Strong Connection Between Oral Health and Overall Health

The link between your mouth and the rest of your body is more profound than many realize. Recent research has uncovered a clear connection between gum disease and several chronic health conditions. This chapter explores how maintaining good oral health can protect and improve your entire body's function.

1. Heart Disease

Your heart is one of your most important organs, and taking care of your mouth can help protect it. Studies have shown that people with gum disease are at a higher risk of developing heart disease. In fact, those with gum disease are **two to three times more likely** to have heart disease.

So, how does this connection work? When gum disease sets in, harmful bacteria from infected gums can enter the bloodstream and travel to the heart. The inflammation caused by these bacteria is thought to contribute to plaque buildup in the arteries (atherosclerosis), which can increase the risk of heart attacks, strokes, and high blood pressure.

Healthy gums are not just about avoiding pain—they are a proactive step toward a healthier cardiovascular system. By maintaining your oral health, you are directly protecting your heart and improving circulation.

2. Diabetes

Oral health and diabetes are tightly connected. People with diabetes are more susceptible to gum disease because the body's immune system is weakened, making it harder to fight infections. Conversely, gum disease can worsen blood sugar control, making it more difficult to manage diabetes.

Treating gum disease can help improve blood sugar control, which is why it's essential to address both conditions as early as possible. By keeping your mouth free of infections, you are making it easier to manage diabetes and reduce the risk of complications.

3. Respiratory Health

The health of your mouth also impacts your lungs. Bacteria from the mouth can enter the bloodstream and travel to the lungs, potentially causing infections such as pneumonia. This is especially true for individuals with chronic respiratory conditions like **COPD (chronic obstructive pulmonary disease)** or weakened immune systems.

Research has found that gum disease can increase the risk of lung infections because bacteria can be inhaled into the respiratory tract. By maintaining good oral hygiene, you can reduce the bacteria in your mouth, helping to lower your risk of respiratory issues and making it easier to breathe.

4. Pregnancy and Birth Outcomes

For women, maintaining good oral health during pregnancy is crucial. Studies have shown that untreated gum disease during pregnancy can increase the risk of preterm birth and low birth weight babies. Women with gum disease are **twice as likely** to give birth prematurely.

The bacteria from gum disease can enter the bloodstream, triggering the release of inflammatory chemicals that may lead to premature labor. Ensuring proper oral care during pregnancy helps protect both the mother and baby's health.

How to Prevent Oral Health Issues and Improve Overall Wellness

The best way to maintain a healthy mouth—and a healthy body—is through prevention. Many oral health issues start small and go unnoticed until they become more serious. This is why regular dental checkups and consistent oral hygiene habits are crucial to keeping both your mouth and body in top shape.

Key Habits for Lifelong Oral Health

1. Brush Properly Twice a Day

Brushing your teeth is the cornerstone of good oral hygiene. However, how you brush matters just as much as how often you do it. Use a soft-bristled toothbrush and fluoride toothpaste, and brush for at least **two minutes** to remove plaque and food particles. Be gentle when brushing to avoid damaging your gums and enamel.

2. Don't Skip Flossing

Flossing is essential for preventing gum disease. It removes food particles and bacteria from areas your toothbrush can't reach—especially between your teeth and below the gumline.

Make flossing a part of your daily routine to keep your gums healthy and reduce the risk of plaque buildup.

3. Watch Your Diet

What you eat affects not only your overall health but also your oral health. Sugary and acidic foods encourage the growth of harmful bacteria in your mouth, leading to cavities and tooth decay. Instead, eat a balanced diet rich in fruits, vegetables, whole grains, and lean proteins. These foods support your body's overall health and help protect your teeth.

4. Drink Plenty of Water

Staying hydrated is important for your overall health—and your oral health. Drinking water helps rinse away food particles and bacteria, keeping your mouth clean. Fluoridated water is especially beneficial, as it helps strengthen your enamel and protect your teeth from decay.

5. Get Regular Dental Checkups

Even if your teeth feel fine, regular dental visits are essential for early detection of problems. During checkups, your dentist can spot early signs of gum disease, cavities, and other oral health issues. Regular visits ensure that your teeth and gums stay healthy and allow for prompt treatment before problems escalate.

Invest in Your Smile, Invest in Your Health

Your smile is not just about aesthetics—it's a reflection of your overall health. By committing to lifelong dental wellness, you are not only protecting your teeth but also your heart, lungs, and even your immune system. Taking simple, consistent steps today can lead to a healthier future.

In the next chapter, we'll explore how to build habits that will keep your teeth healthy for life and help you achieve lasting, optimal oral health.

CHAPTER

II

THE ESSENTIALS OF ORAL HYGIENE

The Science Behind Brushing and Flossing Correctly

Brushing and flossing are simple but essential practices that protect your teeth, gums, and overall health. But have you ever wondered why these two actions are so crucial? The science behind them is straightforward and incredibly important. Let's break it down:

Brushing: The Foundation of Oral Hygiene

Brushing your teeth is a primary defense against plaque buildup, a sticky film of bacteria that naturally forms on your teeth throughout the day. If left unchecked, plaque can lead to gum disease, cavities, and bad breath. Plaque doesn't just cause visible damage—it can affect your body's overall health too.

Brushing does more than just freshen your breath; it removes plaque and bacteria, which can help prevent serious health conditions like heart disease and diabetes.

- **Brush twice a day** for at least two minutes, and make sure to cover all areas of your mouth: front, back, and chewing surfaces.
- **Use a soft-bristled toothbrush**—too firm, and you could damage your gums and enamel.
- **Use gentle, circular motions** instead of aggressive scrubbing, which could irritate your gums and enamel.
- **Fluoride toothpaste** strengthens tooth enamel, helping to prevent cavities and decay. Choose one with the **ADA Seal of Acceptance** to ensure it's effective.

Brushing properly protects your teeth, but there's one area brushing alone can't reach: the space between your teeth.

Flossing: Reaching the Hard-to-Reach Spots

Flossing is often the most neglected part of an oral care routine, but it's crucial for preventing cavities and gum disease. It's the only way to clean between your teeth and along the gumline, where plaque and food particles tend to hide.

- **Floss once a day**, ideally before bedtime, to ensure you've removed the day's buildup.
- **Gently slide the floss between your teeth**, curving it around each tooth to remove plaque and food debris. Avoid snapping the floss as it can irritate your gums.
- **Flossing before brushing** can help remove debris and plaque, making your brushing more effective.

Together, brushing and flossing create a powerful defense against oral health issues, keeping your teeth and gums clean and your body healthier.

Choosing the Right Dental Products

Choosing the right tools can make a big difference in how effectively you maintain your oral hygiene routine. With a wide variety of products on the market, it can be confusing to know where to start. Here are some tips on how to pick the best products for your needs:

Toothbrush: Manual vs. Electric

When it comes to toothbrushes, there's no one-size-fits-all solution. However, research shows that electric toothbrushes tend to remove plaque more effectively than manual ones.

- **Electric toothbrushes**: They make brushing easier and more efficient, especially for people who may struggle to brush thoroughly for two minutes. Look for one with a timer to ensure you brush for the recommended duration.
- **Manual toothbrushes**: As long as you use the proper technique and brush for two minutes, a manual toothbrush can also be effective.

The key is to choose a toothbrush that feels comfortable and allows you to reach all areas of your mouth. Whether electric or manual, always opt for a toothbrush with **soft bristles** to prevent gum irritation and enamel erosion.

Toothpaste: Choose Wisely

While toothpaste is often seen as a simple product, there's a lot to consider. Different toothpastes offer different benefits:

- **Fluoride toothpaste** strengthens tooth enamel and helps prevent cavities. It's a must-have in any oral care routine.

- **Whitening toothpastes** contain mild abrasives to help remove surface stains but should not be relied upon as a primary whitening solution.
- **Sensitivity toothpaste** contains ingredients like potassium nitrate or stannous fluoride to help reduce tooth sensitivity.
- **Gum care toothpastes** are designed to help reduce gum inflammation and improve gum health.

Look for the **ADA Seal of Acceptance** to ensure the toothpaste is effective and safe.

Floss: Which One to Choose?

The type of floss you use can make a big difference in how effective it is at removing plaque.

- **Waxed floss** is smooth and easy to use, especially for tight spaces.
- **Unwaxed floss** is thinner and may be more effective at scraping plaque away but can be harder to maneuver.
- **Floss picks** are convenient for quick clean-ups, but traditional floss often provides a more thorough clean.

Choose the floss that works best for your teeth and your comfort level—just make sure you're using it regularly.

Mouthwash: The Finishing Touch

Mouthwash isn't a replacement for brushing and flossing, but it can be a great addition to your routine. It helps kill bacteria, freshen breath, and reduce plaque buildup.

- **Antiseptic mouthwashes** can help reduce bacteria that contribute to gum disease.

- **Fluoride mouthwashes** can provide extra protection against cavities by strengthening your tooth enamel.
- For dry mouth, use **saliva-stimulating mouthwashes** to keep your mouth moist.

Myths vs. Facts About Oral Hygiene

There are plenty of misconceptions about oral care. Let's bust some of the most common myths and get to the facts.

Myth #1: Brushing harder removes more plaque.

Fact: Brushing too hard can harm your gums and wear down your enamel. The key is to use a **gentle, circular motion** with a soft-bristled toothbrush. This will effectively remove plaque without damaging your gums or teeth.

Myth #2: You only need to floss when something is stuck between your teeth.

Fact: Flossing is essential even if you don't have food stuck between your teeth. Plaque builds up between teeth every day, and flossing is the only way to remove it. Consistent flossing helps prevent gum disease and cavities.

Myth #3: All toothpastes are the same.

Fact: Toothpastes vary widely in terms of what they offer. While fluoride toothpaste is essential, there are specialized options for whitening, sensitivity, gum health, and more. Choose a toothpaste that fits your needs and always check for the **ADA Seal of Acceptance**.

Myth #4: Mouthwash can replace brushing.

Fact: While mouthwash can help freshen your breath and kill bacteria, it cannot replace brushing and flossing. It should be used as a supplement, not a substitute. Brushing and flossing are still your best defense against oral health issues.

Myth #5: Baby teeth don't need to be taken care of because they'll fall out.

Fact: Baby teeth are essential for proper chewing, speech, and the development of permanent teeth. If they're neglected, it can lead to cavities, infections, and alignment issues. Maintaining baby teeth is just as important as caring for adult teeth.

Myth #6: You only need to see a dentist if you have pain or a problem.

Fact: Regular dental checkups are crucial—even if you're not experiencing pain or problems. Many dental issues, like cavities or gum disease, can develop without noticeable symptoms. Early detection is key to preventing more serious issues down the line.

Myth #7: Sugar-free gum is bad for your teeth.

Fact: In fact, **sugar-free gum** can be beneficial for your teeth. It helps stimulate saliva production, which can neutralize acids in the mouth and protect tooth enamel. Choose gum that contains **xylitol**, which has been shown to help prevent cavities.

Myth #8: You should rinse with water after brushing to wash away fluoride.

Fact: Rinsing with water after brushing can wash away the fluoride toothpaste that helps protect your teeth. After brushing, it's best to avoid rinsing immediately. Let the fluoride work its magic and stay on your teeth for longer protection.

Conclusion

Brushing and flossing correctly is the foundation of maintaining a healthy mouth and body. Armed with the right tools and techniques, you can make a significant impact on your oral health. By debunking common myths and sticking to the facts, you'll ensure that your oral hygiene routine is effective in preventing cavities, gum disease, and even more serious health conditions.

In the next chapter, we'll take a closer look at how your diet and lifestyle choices play a pivotal role in supporting your oral health—and how small changes today can lead to lifelong dental wellness.

CHAPTER

III

NUTRITION AND YOUR TEETH

Foods That Strengthen Enamel and Gums

The health of your teeth and gums doesn't just depend on brushing and flossing—it's also deeply influenced by the food you eat. Your mouth needs certain nutrients to fight off decay, strengthen enamel, and support your gums. Eating the right foods can help protect your smile and ensure you maintain oral health well into your later years.

Nutrients Essential for Oral Health

When it comes to protecting your smile, there are a few key nutrients to focus on. These help reinforce your teeth and gums and prevent common dental issues such as tooth decay, gum disease, and enamel erosion.

- **Calcium**: The building block of your teeth and bones, calcium keeps enamel strong and resistant to decay. Without enough calcium, your teeth may become more prone to cavities and sensitivity.

  - **Best sources**: Dairy products like milk, cheese, and yogurt; leafy greens like spinach and kale; almonds and fortified plant-based milks (almond, soy, oat).

- **Vitamin D**: Vitamin D supports your body's ability to absorb calcium, which in turn strengthens your teeth. It also plays a role in reducing inflammation, supporting gum health, and boosting your immune system.

  - **Best sources**: Fatty fish (salmon, mackerel), egg yolks, fortified milk, cereals, and exposure to sunlight.

- **Vitamin C**: Vitamin C is crucial for healthy gums and soft tissue repair. It helps prevent gum disease by supporting collagen production, which strengthens the connective tissues around your teeth.

  - **Best sources**: Citrus fruits (oranges, grapefruit, lemons), bell peppers, strawberries, kiwi, and broccoli.

- **Phosphorus**: This mineral works alongside calcium to maintain strong teeth and bones. Phosphorus also plays an essential role in helping your body use vitamins and minerals more effectively.

  - **Best sources**: Eggs, lean meats, poultry, fish, beans, and nuts.

- **Magnesium**: Magnesium contributes to the health of bones and teeth and helps keep gums firm and healthy. It also works with calcium to build strong enamel.

    - **Best sources**: Whole grains, leafy greens, nuts, seeds, and legumes.
- **Fluoride**: Fluoride is essential for remineralizing your enamel and preventing cavities. It helps neutralize acids in your mouth, making it harder for plaque to build up.

    - **Best sources**: Fluoride toothpaste, and some seafood.
- **Iron**: A lack of iron can contribute to gum disease and tooth loss, as it weakens your immune system and reduces the body's ability to fight infections. It's important to include iron-rich foods in your diet for optimal oral health.

    - **Best sources**: Red meat, poultry, beans, spinach, and fortified cereals.

Foods That Boost Oral Health

Certain foods can offer additional benefits for your teeth. These foods help neutralize acids in the mouth, remove food particles from your teeth, or support saliva production—all of which help reduce the risk of tooth decay and gum disease.

- **Crunchy fruits and vegetables**: Apples, carrots, celery, and cucumbers act as natural toothbrushes by scrubbing your teeth while you chew. They also stimulate saliva production, which helps rinse away bacteria and food particles.
- **Cheese and dairy products**: Cheese, in particular, is great for oral health. It helps raise the pH level in the mouth, which makes it harder for harmful bacteria to thrive. Cheese also contains calcium and phosphorus, which strengthen tooth enamel.
- **Green tea**: Green tea contains polyphenols that reduce harmful bacteria in the mouth, helping to prevent cavities

and gum disease. Drinking unsweetened green tea can help keep your mouth fresh and free of plaque.

- **Nuts and seeds**: These are rich in healthy fats, proteins, and minerals that help protect your teeth. Almonds, walnuts, and sunflower seeds are especially helpful in neutralizing acids and supporting enamel strength.
- **Water**: Staying hydrated is essential for oral health. Water helps wash away food particles, bacteria, and acids, and promotes healthy saliva production. Saliva is your body's natural defense against cavities and gum disease.

Hidden Dangers in Popular Foods and Drinks

While many foods are great for your health, others can significantly damage your teeth. Some foods may seem harmless, but they can lead to plaque buildup, enamel erosion, cavities, and gum disease. Here's a closer look at some of the most common offenders:

The Sugar Problem

Sugar is one of the biggest culprits when it comes to tooth decay. The bacteria in your mouth feed on sugar, producing acids that erode enamel and create cavities. Even foods that aren't overtly sweet can contain sugar and contribute to oral health problems.

- **Sugary drinks**: Soda, sweetened coffee and tea, and fruit juices are all loaded with sugar and acidity. Even 100% fruit juice can be problematic due to its high sugar content and acidity, which can weaken enamel.

- **Processed snacks**: Granola bars, flavored yogurt, and even some "healthy" snack foods often contain added sugars. While they might seem like a good choice, the sugar they contain can lead to cavities if not properly cleaned from your teeth.
- **Candies**: Hard and chewy candies are a double threat to your oral health. They stick to your teeth, providing a constant source of sugar for bacteria, and can also crack or chip teeth if you bite down too hard.

Acidic Foods and Drinks

Acidic foods and beverages can erode enamel over time, making your teeth more susceptible to decay and sensitivity. While citrus fruits and juices are healthy, their high acidity can weaken your enamel if consumed in large amounts.

- **Citrus fruits**: Oranges, lemons, limes, and grapefruits are high in citric acid, which can soften enamel. Consuming them in moderation is key—after eating citrus, rinse your mouth with water to reduce the acidity.
- **Tomato-based foods**: Pasta sauces, salsa, and ketchup are highly acidic. If eaten frequently, they can weaken enamel. After eating these foods, rinse with water to neutralize the acid.
- **Wine**: Both red and white wine are acidic, and the tannins in red wine can stain your teeth. Drinking wine through a straw or rinsing with water afterward can help minimize enamel erosion.

Sticky and Hard Foods

Sticky and hard foods can cause physical damage to your teeth, especially if you're not careful when eating them. These types of foods can also increase your risk for cavities and gum disease.

- **Sticky candies**: Caramel, toffee, gummies, and other chewy treats can stick to your teeth, providing a perfect breeding ground for bacteria.
- **Hard candies**: Sucking on lollipops or hard candies can increase your risk of cavities, and biting them down too forcefully can lead to cracked or chipped teeth.
- **Ice cubes**: Biting down on ice can damage your teeth and lead to cracks or fractures. It's better to avoid chewing on ice altogether.

Tobacco and Alcohol

Both alcohol and tobacco are major risk factors for oral health problems, from tooth decay to oral cancer.

- **Tobacco**: Smoking or chewing tobacco is linked to gum disease, tooth loss, and oral cancer. Tobacco use reduces blood flow to your gums, which weakens your body's ability to fight off infection. It also contributes to bad breath and staining of the teeth.
- **Alcohol**: Alcoholic drinks can cause dry mouth, reducing the amount of saliva in your mouth. Saliva is crucial for neutralizing acids and washing away food particles and bacteria. Alcohol also contributes to gum irritation and an increased risk of oral cancer.

Customized Dietary Advice at Apolonia Smiles

At Apolonia Smiles, we understand that no two people are the same, and that includes their dietary needs. We offer personalized guidance to help you maintain optimal oral health based on your unique lifestyle, preferences, and oral health concerns.

Personalized Nutritional Recommendations

Your oral health journey begins with understanding what your specific needs are. Whether you're trying to reduce plaque buildup, strengthen weakened enamel, or manage gum disease, we'll work with you to create a tailored nutrition plan that suits your goals. We can help you identify foods to include in your diet, as well as those to avoid, ensuring that you give your smile the best chance of staying healthy for life.

Helping You Build Sustainable Habits

Maintaining oral health requires consistency. We'll help you develop long-lasting habits—such as mindful eating and regular hydration—that will protect your teeth and gums every day. We'll also show you how to incorporate foods into your routine that can support your overall health, from boosting immunity to preventing chronic conditions like diabetes and heart disease.

Conclusion

Your diet is one of the most important factors in maintaining healthy teeth and gums. By making smart food choices and incorporating the right nutrients into your daily meals, you can protect your smile, prevent decay, and ensure lifelong oral health. Remember to focus on foods rich in calcium, vitamins, and minerals, while avoiding sugary, acidic, and sticky foods that can harm your enamel.

CHAPTER

IV

PREVENTATIVE DENTISTRY – YOUR BEST INVESTMENT

The Importance of Regular Check-ups and Cleanings

Dental care is often seen as something we only seek when there's pain, discomfort, or an obvious issue. But here's the truth: waiting until something hurts is not the best way to protect your smile or your overall health. In fact, regular dental check-ups and cleanings are one of the smartest and most cost-effective ways to ensure lifelong oral health—and the benefits extend well beyond just your teeth.

Why Regular Visits Matter

1. **Prevent Future Problems**

   Many oral health issues develop slowly, without causing noticeable pain or discomfort at first. Early stages of cavities, gum disease, and even oral cancer can go unnoticed by the patient. Regular dental check-ups help catch these issues while they're still small and easier to treat. This proactive approach prevents future dental problems from becoming bigger, more painful, and expensive to fix.

2. **Professional Cleanings Matter**
   Even if you brush and floss diligently, a toothbrush and floss can't remove everything. Plaque and tartar can build up on teeth and gums over time, even with the best home care. Professional cleanings allow your dentist or hygienist to remove this hardened plaque (tartar) that can't be removed with regular brushing. This helps prevent cavities, gum disease, and even bad breath.
3. **Customized Advice**
   Each person's oral care needs are different. During regular visits, your dentist can assess your unique situation—whether it's cavity-prone teeth, gum sensitivity, or issues like teeth grinding—and offer tailored advice and tips. These personalized recommendations help you maintain your oral health and avoid potential problems.

Early Detection: Catching Issues Before They Escalate

When it comes to oral health, the earlier you catch a problem, the easier and more affordable it is to treat. Early detection is the heart of preventative care.

1. Small Cavities Don't Stay Small

Cavities start small, often without any obvious symptoms, and if left untreated, they can grow into more significant problems. If a cavity is caught early, your dentist can simply fill it. However, if it's left to develop, you may need a root canal or even a crown—both more invasive and expensive procedures. Regular check-ups allow for the early detection of cavities, saving you from these larger issues.

2. Gum Disease Can Be Stopped in Its Tracks

Gum disease is one of the most common causes of tooth loss, but it's also one of the most preventable. Gingivitis, the early stage of gum disease, often doesn't cause pain or noticeable symptoms. However, when caught early, it can usually be reversed with a professional cleaning and improved oral hygiene at home. If left untreated, gingivitis can develop into periodontitis, a much more serious condition that may require surgery or even tooth extraction. Regular dental visits allow your dentist to detect and treat gum disease before it progresses.

3. Oral Cancer Detection

Oral cancer is not something most people think about when they go for a dental check-up, but it's a serious issue. Early detection is key to successful treatment. During your routine check-up, your dentist will examine your mouth for any signs of oral cancer, such as unusual growths, sores, or lesions. If detected early, oral cancer is highly treatable. Regular check-ups increase the chances of catching oral cancer early, potentially saving your life.

How Apolonia Smiles Tailors Prevention Plans for Every Patient

Preventative dentistry is not one-size-fits-all. At Apolonia Smiles, we understand that each patient has unique needs based on their age, lifestyle, and oral health history. We take the time to create a customized prevention plan that helps you achieve optimal oral health—today and for the long term.

Personalized Risk Assessment

When you come in for a check-up, we start by evaluating your individual risk factors. This includes assessing your oral health history, lifestyle (such as diet, tobacco use, or teeth grinding), and any current oral health concerns. Some people are more prone to cavities, while others may have a higher risk of gum disease or tooth sensitivity. By understanding these risks, we can provide tailored recommendations that address your specific needs.

Customized Care Plans

Based on your assessment, we design a care plan that fits your lifestyle. For example, if you're at a higher risk for cavities, we might recommend fluoride treatments to help strengthen your enamel. If gum disease is a concern, we may suggest more frequent cleanings or specific home care tips to keep your gums healthy. Whether you need teeth sealants, whitening advice, or guidance on managing dental anxiety, we're here to help you make informed decisions about your dental health.

Ongoing Monitoring and Adjustments

Your needs may change over time. At each visit, we monitor your oral health and make adjustments to your prevention plan as needed. If we notice signs of gum disease or early tooth decay, we'll address them before they turn into bigger problems. We believe that taking a proactive approach to your oral care ensures that you can avoid costly treatments down the line and enjoy a healthy smile for a lifetime.

How Preventative Dentistry Saves You Money in the Long Run

Preventative care is not only about keeping your smile looking great—it's also a wise financial decision. Regular check-ups and cleanings can help you avoid major dental procedures down the road, which can be expensive and time-consuming.

1. **Less Expensive Treatments**
   Catching a problem early means less invasive treatment, which often costs less. For example, filling a small cavity is much more affordable than needing a root canal or crown. By staying on top of your dental visits, you avoid these larger, more costly procedures.
2. **Prevent Tooth Loss**
   Gum disease and tooth decay are leading causes of tooth loss. Losing a tooth, or several, can be costly to replace with implants, bridges, or dentures. Regular dental visits can help you maintain a full, healthy set of teeth for years to come.
3. **Improved Overall Health**
   The benefits of good oral health extend far beyond your mouth. Maintaining healthy teeth and gums can help lower your risk of serious health conditions like heart disease, diabetes, and respiratory issues. Preventing these problems in the first place can save you money on medical bills down the road.

Conclusion: Invest in Your Smile for a Lifetime

Investing in preventative dentistry is one of the best decisions you can make for both your smile and your health. By attending regular check-ups, receiving professional cleanings, and working with your dentist to create a personalized prevention plan, you're not only protecting your teeth, but you're also reducing the risk of more serious health issues. At Apolonia Smiles, we're committed to helping you achieve lifelong dental wellness through prevention.

Remember, your smile is one of your most valuable assets—take care of it now to enjoy a lifetime of health and confidence. In the next chapter, we'll dive into restorative dentistry and how it can help you address any issues that arise, restoring both the function and beauty of your smile.

CHAPTER

V

RESTORATIVE DENTISTRY – REBUILDING CONFIDENCE

When it comes to your smile, sometimes things don't go as planned. Teeth can get damaged, worn down, or even lost. The good news? Restorative dentistry offers a range of effective treatments designed to restore the function and appearance of your teeth, giving you the confidence to smile freely again.

Modern Solutions for Cavities, Cracks, and Missing Teeth

Restorative dentistry is all about fixing and rebuilding teeth that have been damaged, decayed, or lost. Whether it's a small cavity or a significant loss of teeth, restorative treatments offer a way to recover your smile's functionality and beauty. Here's a look at some of the most common dental issues and the solutions that can help:

1. **Cavities**

Cavities, or dental decay, are a common issue, but they don't have to be a lifelong problem. If caught early, a cavity can be treated with a simple filling. Modern materials, such as tooth-colored composites, not only restore the tooth's shape but also blend seamlessly with your natural teeth. These fillings are strong, durable, and give your smile a natural, healthy appearance.

2. **Cracked or Broken Teeth**

   Whether caused by an accident, chewing hard food, or the wear of everyday life, cracked or broken teeth are another common issue. The good news is that there are several ways to fix cracked or broken teeth without sacrificing aesthetics. Depending on the severity, your dentist may recommend solutions like crowns or bonding. These restorations can help protect and restore your tooth, making it functional and healthy once more.

3. **Missing Teeth**

   Losing a tooth—whether from injury, decay, or gum disease—can have a significant impact on both your appearance and your overall health. Missing teeth make chewing and speaking difficult and can cause the surrounding teeth to shift, affecting your bite. Fortunately, restorative dentistry offers several options to replace missing teeth and restore your smile.

The Role of Implants, Crowns, and Bridges in Restoring Your Smile

Restorative dentistry offers several options to address tooth loss, and each solution comes with its own benefits. Here's a closer look at three common restorative treatments: dental implants, crowns, and bridges.

1. **Dental Implants – A Permanent Solution to Missing Teeth**

   When it comes to replacing missing teeth, dental implants are one of the most advanced and reliable options available. Unlike traditional dentures or bridges, implants are permanently placed into your jawbone, acting as a substitute for the root of the missing tooth. A small titanium post is surgically inserted into the bone, and over time, it fuses with the bone in a process known as osseointegration. Once the implant has securely bonded with the bone, a custom-made crown is attached, providing a durable and natural-looking replacement tooth.

   The advantages of dental implants are numerous. They're the most natural-looking and feeling option for replacing a missing tooth. Implants also help preserve the bone structure of your jaw, preventing the bone loss that typically occurs after tooth loss. Additionally, because the implant is securely anchored, you don't have to worry about slippage or discomfort, which can sometimes occur with dentures or bridges. Implants can also be used to support multiple teeth, making them an ideal choice for larger gaps or even full arch restorations.

2. **Crowns – Protecting Damaged Teeth**

   Dental crowns are used to cover and protect teeth that have been extensively damaged or weakened due to decay, cracks, or large fillings. A crown acts as a cap that encases the tooth, restoring its size, shape, and function. Crowns are often made from porcelain or ceramic, materials that mimic the look of natural teeth, so your restoration will blend seamlessly with your smile.

   Crowns are typically used after a root canal treatment or for severely damaged teeth. They provide strength and protection, ensuring the tooth remains functional for years to come.

3. **Bridges – Filling the Gaps Left by Missing Teeth**
A dental bridge is another option for replacing missing teeth, especially when there are adjacent healthy teeth to support it. A bridge consists of one or more artificial teeth, anchored in place by crowns placed on the neighboring teeth. Bridges restore both the appearance and function of your smile, helping you chew, speak, and smile with confidence.

Why Implants Stand Out in Restorative Dentistry

Dental implants have revolutionized restorative dentistry. They're widely considered the gold standard for replacing missing teeth, offering several advantages over other options:

- **Natural Appearance**: Implants are designed to look, feel, and function just like your natural teeth. Unlike dentures, which can shift in the mouth, implants stay securely in place, offering a more natural and comfortable experience.
- **Long-Lasting Solution**: Implants are incredibly durable and can last a lifetime with proper care. Because the implant fuses with your jawbone, it becomes a permanent part of your mouth, unlike bridges or dentures, which may need to be replaced after a certain period.
- **Improved Oral Health**: Since implants are placed directly into the jawbone, they help preserve bone density. Missing teeth can lead to bone loss in the jaw, but implants stimulate the bone, preventing further deterioration. This

helps maintain the structure of your face and jaw, keeping you looking younger for longer.

- **No Need for Adjacent Tooth Modifications**: Unlike bridges, which require shaving down the neighboring teeth to accommodate crowns, implants don't affect adjacent teeth. This means more of your natural teeth remain intact.

If you're missing one or more teeth, dental implants may be the ideal solution for restoring your smile and oral health. They provide a secure, natural-looking, and long-term solution to tooth loss, helping you regain your confidence and quality of life.

The Emotional Impact of Restorative Dentistry

Restorative dentistry is about more than just restoring the physical function of your teeth. It's also about rebuilding confidence and improving your overall well-being. Having a full, healthy smile can significantly enhance your self-esteem, social interactions, and even your career. People with missing or damaged teeth often feel self-conscious, which can affect their confidence in both personal and professional situations.

With the help of restorative treatments like dental implants, crowns, and bridges, you can restore your smile—and your confidence—without compromising on quality or comfort. Whether you've lost a tooth due to decay, injury, or aging, restorative dentistry has the solutions to help you smile brighter and live better.

CHAPTER

VI

COSMETIC DENTISTRY – ENHANCING YOUR SMILE

Your smile is far more than just a feature of your face—it's an expression of your personality, your confidence, and your overall well-being. When you smile, you not only brighten up the room, but you also send a positive signal to the people around you. Cosmetic dentistry offers transformative options to help you achieve a smile that reflects the best version of yourself, inside and out.

Teeth Whitening – A Fresh Start for Your Smile

Over time, teeth naturally become stained or discolored due to food, drinks, smoking, or even just the aging process. While maintaining excellent oral hygiene can help prevent staining, some discoloration is inevitable. Teeth whitening is one of the most effective ways to restore brightness and radiance to your smile.

Professional whitening treatments, unlike over-the-counter products, are customized to your needs and can dramatically improve the appearance of your teeth in a short amount of time. In-office whitening can provide immediate, stunning results, while take-home options allow for a gradual but noticeable improvement in the comfort of your own home.

A brighter smile not only enhances your appearance but can also help boost your mood and confidence. It's an easy and non-invasive way to make your smile appear younger, healthier, and more vibrant.

Veneers – Perfecting Your Smile, One Tooth at a Time

Veneers are thin, custom-designed shells that cover the front surfaces of your teeth. They're ideal for correcting imperfections such as chips, cracks, severe staining, or minor misalignment. For patients looking for a complete makeover or a subtle improvement, veneers offer the perfect balance of aesthetic beauty and long-lasting durability.

Made from high-quality porcelain or resin composite, veneers mimic the natural translucency and strength of real teeth. They're tailored to fit seamlessly with the contours of your smile, ensuring a completely natural look that enhances your overall facial features.

Veneers are incredibly versatile. They can address a variety of dental concerns at once—creating a smooth, uniform appearance for your smile. With proper care, veneers can last for years, making them a lasting investment in your self-confidence and overall appearance.

Smile Makeovers – Comprehensive Transformation

A smile makeover is a comprehensive, individualized approach to enhancing your smile through multiple cosmetic procedures. It's ideal for patients who want to address several aspects of their smile at once, whether that includes whitening, reshaping, bonding, or using veneers and crowns. A smile makeover is not just about aesthetics; it's about creating a smile that complements your natural facial features while improving the function and health of your teeth.

Because each patient is unique, a smile makeover is fully personalized. Your dentist will assess your oral health, discuss your goals, and design a plan that aligns with your vision of an ideal smile. This holistic approach ensures that your smile makeover is more than just a quick fix—it's a transformation that lasts.

Incorporating various treatments in a smile makeover offers multiple benefits. From subtle improvements to dramatic changes, the result is a harmonious, balanced smile that makes you feel great about how you look, and more confident in how you present yourself to the world.

The Power of a Smile in Your Personal and Professional Life

A smile is not only an asset in social interactions, but it also holds powerful significance in your career and personal relationships. In many ways, your smile serves as a gateway to the first impression you make on others. A confident smile exudes warmth, friendliness, and approachability, all of which are critical traits in building connections, whether in casual settings or business environments.

Studies have shown that people who smile often are perceived as more trustworthy, approachable, and confident. Smiling can leave a positive impression, leading to better social interactions, improved relationships, and even professional success. Whether you're at a job interview, meeting new clients, or making an important presentation, a beautiful smile can elevate your presence and help you stand out for all the right reasons.

Moreover, having a smile that you're proud of can improve how you feel about yourself. When you're confident in your smile, you're more likely to express yourself freely, engage with others openly, and be your authentic self. Cosmetic dentistry not only transforms how others perceive you, but it also empowers you to be more confident in your own skin.

The Life-Changing Impact of a Beautiful Smile

Cosmetic dentistry offers more than just aesthetic benefits—it also plays an important role in your overall well-being. When you feel good about the way you look, it improves your self-esteem, reduces anxiety in social situations, and gives you the freedom to smile without hesitation. A beautiful smile is often the first step in a journey toward better self-care, greater confidence, and more meaningful connections with the world around you.

Many of our patients have experienced not just an improvement in their smile, but a positive shift in how they feel about themselves. A radiant smile can boost your mood and energy levels, as well as influence your interactions in more powerful and meaningful ways.

Customized Cosmetic Treatments for Every Patient

Cosmetic dentistry is deeply personalized. It's not just about changing the appearance of your teeth—it's about understanding what makes your smile unique and how to enhance that uniqueness to meet your personal goals. Whether you want a subtle adjustment or a complete smile makeover, cosmetic dentistry offers a variety of treatment options that can be tailored to your specific needs.

During your consultation, your dentist will take the time to understand your expectations and help guide you through the various options available. From teeth whitening to veneers, crowns, or even full smile makeovers, the goal is always to create a smile that reflects the best version of you. You'll work closely with your dentist to design a treatment plan that's right for you—one that enhances both the health and aesthetics of your smile.

Your smile is a reflection of your identity. Cosmetic dentistry helps ensure that it's a smile you'll love, one that serves you throughout your life, and one that enhances your natural beauty with lasting results.

Investing in Your Smile for the Future

A beautiful smile is an investment that will pay off in many ways for years to come. It's not just about looking good in the moment, but about creating long-term benefits for your confidence, health, and overall well-being. Whether you choose whitening treatments, veneers, or a complete smile makeover, cosmetic dentistry offers the opportunity to improve your appearance, boost your self-esteem, and elevate your quality of life.

When you invest in your smile, you're investing in yourself. With the help of your dentist, you can create a smile that not only looks great but also complements your life's goals and ambitions. Your smile is a reflection of who you are and who you strive to be—it's time to make sure it's the best it can be.

CHAPTER

VII

ORTHODONTICS – MORE THAN JUST STRAIGHT TEETH

When most people think of orthodontics, they picture braces or clear aligners used to straighten teeth. While improving your smile's appearance is a key benefit of orthodontic treatment, it's only part of the story. Orthodontics can have a profound impact on your overall dental health, function, and comfort, and the benefits go far beyond just aesthetics.

The Benefits of Clear Aligners and Braces Beyond Aesthetics

1. Improved Functionality: Straight teeth do more than look good—they also function better. When your teeth are properly aligned, you can chew more effectively and with less strain on your jaw muscles. Misaligned teeth can contribute to issues like teeth grinding, jaw pain, and difficulty chewing. Correcting alignment with braces or clear aligners can alleviate these issues, ensuring better oral function.

2. Enhanced Oral Health: Teeth that are out of alignment are harder to clean properly. Over time, this can lead to plaque buildup, gum disease, and tooth decay. When your teeth are aligned, it's easier to brush and floss effectively, reducing the likelihood of cavities and gum problems. Proper alignment also prevents excessive wear on certain teeth caused by misalignment, which can lead to chipped or cracked teeth.

3. Preventing Future Dental Issues: Orthodontic treatments can correct bite issues such as overbite, underbite, crossbite, and open bite. These problems can lead to uneven wear on your teeth, temporomandibular joint (TMJ) disorders, and even sleep apnea. By addressing alignment early, orthodontics can prevent these serious dental problems from developing down the road.

4. Boost in Confidence and Self-Esteem: While the functional and health benefits are important, one of the most significant advantages of orthodontics is the boost in confidence that comes with a straighter smile. Having a smile you feel proud of can have a lasting effect on your self-esteem and social interactions.

The Link Between Alignment and Long-Term Dental Health

Orthodontics isn't just about a beautiful smile—it's an investment in your long-term dental health. Crooked teeth can cause significant strain on your jaw and affect the way your teeth come together, leading to problems like misaligned bites, TMJ disorders, and even tooth loss in severe cases.

For instance, a misaligned bite can lead to excessive wear and tear on certain teeth, which can eventually cause enamel erosion or tooth fractures. Addressing these issues through orthodontics ensures a smoother bite and reduces the strain on individual teeth.

Moreover, properly aligned teeth can reduce the risk of gum disease and tooth decay. When teeth are positioned well, it's easier to maintain oral hygiene, decreasing the chances of plaque buildup and cavities. So, by investing in orthodontics, you're not just straightening your teeth, but also setting up a strong foundation for a lifetime of good oral health.

CHAPTER

VIII

DENTAL ANXIETY AND PAIN-FREE DENTISTRY

It's completely natural to feel anxious about going to the dentist. For many, even the thought of an upcoming dental appointment can cause a sense of dread or worry. Whether it's the fear of pain, the sounds of dental tools, or the simple uncertainty of the unknown, dental anxiety is something that many patients experience. But here's the good news: modern dentistry has evolved in remarkable ways, and there's no reason for you to suffer in silence any longer. Today's dental care is more comfortable, more empathetic, and designed to make your experience as easy and stress-free as possible.

Acknowledging Your Feelings: You Are Not Alone

We understand that dental anxiety is a very real concern, and we want to assure you that you're not alone. Many people—whether it's their first visit or after many years of dental care—feel some form of nervousness when visiting the dentist. You might worry about the procedure itself, or you might feel uneasy about being in a clinical setting. Whatever the cause, these feelings are completely valid, and we respect them.

At Apolonia Smiles, we don't just see you as a patient with teeth to treat—we see you as a person. Your feelings are important, and we're here to listen to your concerns and address them with the utmost compassion. The first step toward a stress-free dental experience is making sure you feel heard, understood, and in control of your care.

We are committed to providing an environment where you can relax and feel safe. You're in good hands, and we'll work with you to find ways to make your visits as calm and comfortable as possible.

How Modern Dentistry Makes Procedures More Comfortable

The advancements in dental care over the past few years are truly remarkable. Treatments that once felt like daunting or painful experiences have been transformed into smooth, almost painless procedures. With cutting-edge technology and modern techniques, you can expect a more comfortable, less stressful visit to the dentist.

1. Advanced Anesthetics

Modern anesthetics are designed to make your treatment as pain-free as possible. We use faster-acting, more effective numbing agents that ensure you remain completely comfortable throughout your procedure. Whether you're having a routine cleaning or something more complex, we will ensure that you are fully numbed before we begin, so you feel no discomfort during treatment.

2. Laser Dentistry

Laser technology has revolutionized the way we perform many dental procedures. Laser dentistry is not only more precise, but it also reduces the discomfort associated with traditional tools. For procedures like cavity fillings, soft tissue treatments, and gum care, lasers are gentle and effective, meaning less vibration, less noise, and a quicker recovery time. There's no need for the traditional drill, which means less anxiety for you.

3. Minimally Invasive Techniques

With the latest tools, our team can perform dental procedures with minimal disruption to surrounding tissue. By using less invasive techniques, we reduce the need for stitches, decrease recovery times, and minimize discomfort. Whether it's filling a cavity or treating gum disease, these modern approaches focus on preserving your natural tooth structure, which helps you heal faster and with less pain.

The Importance of Communication: You Have a Voice

It's easy to feel like you're powerless when you're sitting in the dental chair, but you are in control of your experience. We're here to help you feel confident and calm, and we encourage open communication at every stage of your visit. If you're feeling nervous or unsure about a procedure, please don't hesitate to let us know. We will take the time to explain everything, answer your questions, and ensure you feel fully informed.

We also understand that the unknown can be a major source of anxiety. That's why we make it a priority to explain each step of your treatment plan in clear, straightforward terms. By understanding what to expect, you'll feel more in control, and your worries will begin to fade away.

It's Okay to Feel Anxious—You're Not Alone

We want to remind you that it's okay to feel nervous or anxious about dental visits—it's a completely natural response. You're not alone in this, and there is absolutely no shame in feeling uncertain. What's important is that you're taking steps toward caring for your health, and that's something to be proud of.

At Apolonia Smiles, we believe that your dental care journey is a partnership. You're not just a patient in a chair; you're someone we genuinely care about. Our team is here to support you every step of the way, and we are committed to ensuring that your experience is as pleasant and stress-free as possible. Whether it's your first visit or your fiftieth, we're here to make you feel comfortable, informed, and cared for. You deserve to feel at ease, and we're here to help make that happen.

CHAPTER

IX

THE POWER OF HABIT: MAINTAINING LIFELONG WELLNESS

Developing and maintaining healthy habits is one of the most powerful tools you can use to ensure a lifetime of dental health. But as we all know, habits are not always easy to form. Whether it's exercise, eating well, or brushing and flossing your teeth, we can all face challenges when trying to stick to healthy routines. The good news is that you can leverage the science of habit formation to make dental care a consistent part of your life, so you don't have to think twice about it.

In this chapter, we'll explore how the science of habit can help you maintain a beautiful, healthy smile for life, as well as the importance of regular dental visits and the exclusive wellness programs offered at Apolonia Smiles that support you every step of the way.

The Psychology of Habit: Building Consistency with Dental Care

As Charles Duhigg explains in *The Power of Habit*, habits are formed through a cycle of cues, routines, and rewards. Understanding this cycle is key to transforming your dental care routine into a lasting habit.

- **Cue**: This is the trigger that prompts you to take action. For brushing your teeth, the cue could be waking up in the morning, finishing a meal, or getting ready for bed. Once you become aware of these cues, you can begin to attach them to your new routine.
- **Routine**: This is the behavior you perform when you encounter the cue. In the case of oral hygiene, the routine is brushing, flossing, and using mouthwash.
- **Reward**: The positive feeling you get after completing the routine reinforces the behavior, helping to make it a habit. In dental care, the reward is not just the fresh feeling in your mouth but the long-term benefits, such as fewer cavities, better breath, and healthier gums.

By intentionally setting up cues and rewards, you can make dental care an ingrained part of your daily routine. It may take time, but as with any habit, the more consistent you are, the easier it becomes.

How to Create and Maintain Consistent Dental Care Habits

Consistency is key to building lasting habits—and dental care is no exception. To set yourself up for success, here are a few proven strategies to make maintaining your smile a breeze:

1. **Start Small and Build Gradually**
   Trying to completely overhaul your dental care habits overnight can be overwhelming. Instead, start with small steps, such as committing to brush your teeth every morning and night for a week. As this becomes second nature, slowly add in flossing or using mouthwash. Gradually increasing your routine helps you build a sustainable habit without feeling overwhelmed.
2. **Tie Dental Care to Existing Routines**
   One of the most effective ways to build a habit is by attaching it to something you already do regularly. For example, if you always have a cup of coffee first thing in the morning, try brushing your teeth right after. Linking your dental care to a well-established part of your routine makes it easier to remember and less likely to be skipped.
3. **Track Your Progress and Stay Accountable**
   Research shows that tracking your progress can make a big difference in habit formation. Keep a calendar or use an app to track your brushing, flossing, and dental check-ups. The act of checking off each day can boost your motivation and help you stay consistent.
4. **Celebrate Your Wins**
   Positive reinforcement is an important part of habit-building. Reward yourself for sticking to your dental care routine. It doesn't have to be a big reward—maybe a relaxing evening or a small treat. Celebrating small successes along the way strengthens your commitment to long-term dental health.

The Importance of Regular Dental Visits: Consistency in Professional Care

As important as your daily dental habits are, they can't replace the expertise of a dental professional. Routine check-ups, cleanings, and preventive care are essential to maintaining a healthy smile. Regular visits to the dentist not only ensure your teeth are in good shape, but they also give us the opportunity to detect any potential issues before they become serious problems.

1. **Preventive Care: The Power of Early Detection**
   One of the most significant benefits of regular dental check-ups is early detection. Minor problems, such as small cavities or gum inflammation, can be detected early and treated before they escalate into larger, more costly issues. Regular visits help ensure that you stay ahead of potential oral health problems.
2. **Professional Cleanings: Removing Plaque and Tartar**
   Even with the best at-home care, plaque and tartar can accumulate over time. Professional cleanings are the most effective way to remove this buildup, reducing your risk of cavities and gum disease. Cleanings also give your dentist the chance to assess your oral health and offer personalized advice based on your individual needs.
3. **Personalized Care Plans for Long-Term Success**
   At Apolonia Smiles, we don't believe in one-size-fits-all solutions. Our team will work with you to create a personalized dental care plan tailored to your specific needs and goals. Whether you're looking to improve your gum health, enhance your smile with cosmetic treatments, or simply maintain your oral health, we're here to provide guidance and support every step of the way.

Exclusive Wellness Programs at Apolonia Smiles: Making Your Healthy Habits Rewarding

We know that making and sticking to habits can be challenging, especially when life gets busy. That's why Apolonia Smiles has developed exclusive wellness programs designed to support you in your commitment to long-term dental health. These programs not only help you stay on track with your dental care but also offer rewards for maintaining a consistent routine.

1. **Gentle Reminders for Your Appointments**
   Life gets hectic, and it's easy to forget when your next dental check-up or cleaning is due. At Apolonia Smiles, we send you gentle reminders via text or email so you never miss an appointment. These reminders take the stress out of managing your appointments and help ensure you stay consistent with your oral health care.
2. **Customized Health Plans for Your Lifestyle**
   Our wellness programs go beyond just scheduling check-ups. We work with you to understand your unique lifestyle and oral health needs. Whether you're managing a busy work schedule, dealing with specific oral health concerns, or simply need tips to improve your dental care routine, we provide personalized guidance and support that fits into your life.
3. **Loyalty Rewards and Incentives**
   Sticking to a dental care routine has its rewards—literally! Our wellness programs offer exclusive benefits like discounts on dental services, special promotions, and loyalty rewards for patients who stay consistent with their care. We believe in celebrating your commitment to your oral health and want to make sure you feel supported in every way.

Maintaining Your Smile for Life: The Role of Habits in Your Oral Health Journey

The key to a lifetime of healthy teeth and gums isn't just in occasional treatments or high-tech procedures—it's in the daily habits you form and maintain. By making small, manageable changes to your routine, tracking your progress, and sticking to a schedule of regular dental visits, you can enjoy long-term dental health with ease.

Remember, it's the small, consistent actions that make all the difference. With Apolonia Smiles by your side, we're here to ensure you have all the support, guidance, and rewards you need to build healthy dental habits that will last a lifetime. Together, we can make your smile shine bright for many years to come.

CONCLUSION

Your smile is far more than just a reflection of your teeth—it's a reflection of your health, your confidence, and the care you give to yourself. It's the first thing people often notice, and it's one of the most powerful aspects of your identity. Throughout this book, we've explored the steps to nurturing your smile and maintaining lifelong dental wellness. But, in truth, it's not just about teeth. It's about creating habits, building confidence, and investing in yourself—your smile becomes a legacy that speaks to the care you've taken for your overall health and well-being.

Taking Charge of Your Dental Wellness

Now that you have the knowledge, you have the power to take charge of your dental wellness. Each step you take to care for your smile not only strengthens your oral health, but it supports your overall health as well. Small, consistent actions—like brushing, flossing, and attending regular check-ups—add up over time and lead to lasting results. By embracing these habits and staying committed to self-care, you're building a future of health that goes beyond just your teeth.

Remember, consistency is key. Even when life gets busy, taking time to care for your smile is an investment in yourself. The habits you form today will shape the future of your health and well-being.

Apolonia Smiles: A Partner in Your Journey to Wellness

At Apolonia Smiles, we are dedicated to your complete wellness, not just your smile. We recognize that each person's dental journey is unique, and our commitment is to help you navigate yours with compassion, expertise, and personalized care. Whether you are coming in for a routine check-up, looking to restore your smile, or seeking advanced treatments, we're here to support you with care tailored to your needs.

We aim to build lasting relationships with our patients, creating a space where you feel heard, valued, and empowered. Our team is here not just to treat your teeth, but to help you feel confident, comfortable, and supported throughout your journey.

An Invitation to Begin Your Journey with Us

If you're ready to take the next step, we invite you to schedule a personalized consultation with us. Together, we'll discuss your unique needs and goals, and create a customized plan to ensure your smile remains healthy, vibrant, and an important part of your life for years to come.

Your smile is your legacy, and we're honored to help you protect and enhance it. At Apolonia Smiles, we're not just taking care of your teeth—we're here to help you feel your best and live your healthiest life. We look forward to partnering with you on your journey to lifelong dental wellness.

Thank you for trusting us to be part of your health journey. Your smile will always be worth the investment.

www.ingramcontent.com/pod-product-compliance
Lightning Source LLC
LaVergne TN
LVHW022029200926
848481LV00007B/2609